10,000 STEPS: WALKING FOR WEIGHT LOSS AND HEALTH

A TURN BY TURN ROADMAP

By Ryan J. S. Martin

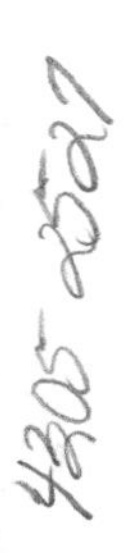

First Printing: 2015
Bright Ideas Editorial
PO Box 4095
Crested Butte, CO 81224
https://www.facebook.com/brightideaseditoria

Disclaimer

Although the author and publisher have made every effort to ensure that the information in this book was correct at press time, the author and publisher do not assume and hereby disclaim any liability to any party for any loss, damage, or disruption caused by errors or omissions, whether such errors or omissions result from negligence, accident, or any other cause.

This book is not intended as a substitute for the medical advice of physicians. The reader should regularly consult a physician in matters relating to his/her health and particularly with respect to any symptoms that may require diagnosis or medical attention.

FREE DOWNLOAD

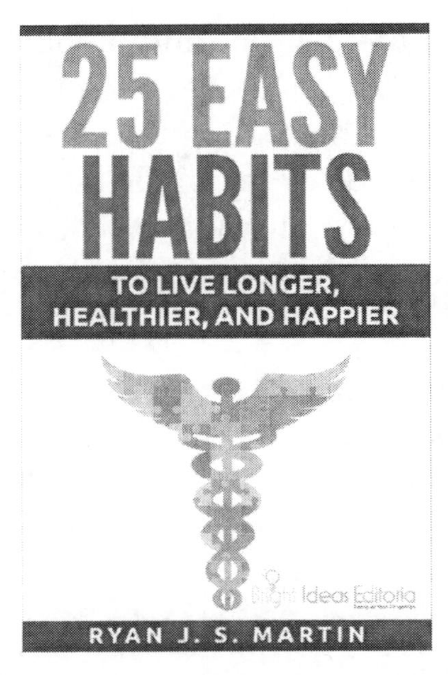

As a way of thanking you for purchasing this book, I am offering a special gift to my readers. This book is not available for purchase anywhere. You can only get it by clicking on the link below.

The power of habit is life altering. Smaller habits are easier to start and stop, and they can have measurable effects in the quality of a person's life. Smaller habits, once formed, grow into larger ones.

Habits can affect your body, your mind, and your spirit. They govern your interactions with friends and family. They control how you work and play. They form the basis for your success and failures.

Whether you have big changes you are ready to make in your life or just want to fine-tune small behaviors, this book can make a difference.

You can download the free book at

https://editoria.leadpages.net/25habits/

Contents

Introduction

> "My grandmother started walking five miles a day when she was sixty. She's ninety-seven now, and we don't know where the hell she is."
>
> Ellen DeGeneres

I bought a new cell phone last spring, and the thing immediately began sending me messages. "Keep it up! You are halfway to your goal!" My what? Without my express invitation, the Activity Zone app had put me on a workout plan. Did it notice the double chins in my selfies? Sense some extra padding through my pocket? Whatever the impetus, my phone was using a built-in motion sensor to track my daily movement, cheering me on to reach 10,000 steps every day.

I don't like to be told what to do, especially by an appliance, but dang if my competitive (obsessive?) genes didn't kick in. I started finding ways to up my step count. I'd take my phone everywhere, even into the bathroom to make sure it recorded each and every move I made. If I forgot to take it somewhere, I'd shake it until it racked up the steps I had missed. My record came last September, the day I took my kids to Disneyland: 30,739 steps. I can't swear that the shaking motion of the rides didn't artificially inflate the count, and frankly, I don't want to know. I'm proud of that record. And I felt three days' worth of tired by the end.

Just to egg me on, the app has assigned me with an international ranking. I am officially 327,915th in the world. If that isn't sufficiently impressive (and who wouldn't be proud to be in the top half-million), I am 62,832nd in my age group. In the past year, I have walked 3,650,411 steps, or 1825 miles, about the distance from Las Vegas to Chicago. Sadly, my step total is but a rounding error compared to the "World's Best." Numero Uno has walked 37,774,447 steps or 18,887 miles, about the same distance from Mexico City to the middle of Alaska. And back. Twice.

That individual, of course, is an extreme. When I scroll through all the rankings, it becomes clear that if the users of this phone represent a random population sampling, then the majority of people old enough to have their own cell phone aren't walking 10,000 steps every day. Not even close. And while it is possible that the data is skewed, that maybe fit people are less likely to let their cell phones boss them around and publish data without their informed consent, I don't really think that is the case. Just by looking at the popularity of diets and weight loss products that promise quick solutions, it is easy to see that millions of people want to be healthier. They just don't want to kill themselves to get that way. Enter walking, stage right

If the average person has a stride length of 2.5 feet, then 10,000 steps is just short of 5 miles. That same average person walking 10,000 steps every day will burn 3500 calories each week, or one pound of body fat. That can really add up over time.

What makes walking for weight loss so appealing, is that is just isn't that hard to do. Anyone who can walk can do it. It is scalable; you can make it as easy or as challenging as you like. You can work it in throughout your day instead of having to dedicate a large block of time to a workout. It doesn't cost anything outside of a good pair of walking shoes and a pedometer. And the benefits extend beyond the physical. Walking relieves stress, helps with depression, and promotes creative thinking too.

This book will take you through the health benefits of walking and show you how to track them. It will give you ways to add more steps to your day, help you find methods to stay motivated, and give you a few tips on keeping yourself safe and free from injury.

Walking is one of the best ways to improve health and lose weight over time. It resets the body and the mind. To take the first step on your journey of 10,000, read on. You could be in San Francisco by Christmas.

Chapter 1: Why Walk 10,000 Steps?

> "I have two doctors, my left leg and my right. When body and mind are out of gear (and those twin parts of me live at such close quarters that the one always catches melancholy from the other) I know that I have only to call in my doctors and I shall be well again." George M. Trevelyan, from *Walking*

More than 5% of all of the books for sale on Amazon fall under the heading of Health, Fitness and Dieting. This is far and away the largest nonfiction category, larger than finance, or relationships or technology. It shows that people feel less in control of their health than any other area of their lives. And it is no wonder. By so many accounts, the American system of health care is broken, and massive government intervention has so far failed to fix it. It is up to the individual to take control of his or her own health and become their own loudest advocate. Just as homeowners need to lock their doors and perhaps install other security measures to protect their property from theft and destruction, people know that they are in charge of guarding against the top two killers, heart disease and cancer. Maintaining a healthy weight and fitness level is a critical part of the plan. As our own champions, we examine all the new information, mostly in the form of popular diets, for solutions.

Many diets promise immediate weight loss results. Many doctors advise losing weight slowly over time by eating healthier and incorporating more exercise. I don't know about you, but I have never purposely bought a slow car, stood in the longest line, or used dial-up internet when high-speed connections were available. And yet, lots of people have lost weight quickly using one method or another, and then gained it back because they were not inspired to stick with their lifestyle changes. Sometimes the meandering, scenic route can be the most fulfilling after all.

The hardest part about starting a new exercise routine is, well, starting it. The journey of a thousand miles and all that. And inevitably, the more out of shape one is, and the more that person's body could benefit from the exercise, the more difficult it is to do the exercises. The exercise gods have an acute sense of irony.

There is a common myth that it takes twenty-one days to form a new habit. Oh, if only that were so. In a blog article called *How Long Does it Actually Take to Form a Habit (Backed by Science)*, James Clear gives some history on this misconception. This idea of forming habits in three weeks, Clear says, started with a plastic surgeon in the 1950s named Maxwell Maltz. Dr. Maltz noticed that it took his patients an average of three weeks to adjust to their altered appearances. He published his observations, and self-help gurus extrapolated this data to mean that all new behavior can become normal in 21 days. More recent studies that followed people who have adopted new positive behaviors found that it actually takes humans an average of 66 days for a habit to become routine.[1] That is more than three times longer than held by conventional wisdom.

When we apply the 66-day results to working out, it becomes obvious why it is so easy to fail. Not only do you have to do something that is difficult on the magnitude of the Seven Labors of Hercules, you have to do it for nine weeks until it becomes the norm. But walking, that is something you already do to one extent or another. The new behavior is in *increasing what you are already doing,* rather than starting something new. The threshold for starting is smaller. Once you get a baseline of the number of steps you currently walk every day, you can gradually ratchet it up until you reach a constant 10,000.

---

[1] http://jamesclear.com/new-habit

Where did the number 10,000 come from? It was an advertising gimmick by Japanese pedometer makers in the 1960s, and the idea stuck around. The CDC recommends getting in a minimum of 150 minutes of moderate activity each week[2], which breaks down to around 8,000 steps each day. But it doesn't hurt to aim higher. If you add in more steps for walking to work, getting around the store, and getting around the house, you end up with a nice round 10,000 steps.

Of course, any of the extra activity that you are able to get into the day is going to improve your health. If you are only able to get 5000 steps in when you start, increasing just by 1000 steps is going to make a big difference. Start slowly and increase to where you would like to be. If you increase above 10,000 steps each day that only means that you have more benefits for your health.

So what are these many health benefits that walking so grandly promises? Actually, a surprising number for both your body and your mind.

Health Benefits

Walking is one of the best exercises for your body because it is easy on your joints, and you can scale both your intensity level and how far and long you walk. Everyone who is able to get up, no matter their health levels, can do it and have fun. Here is a breakdown of some of the benefits:

---

[2] http://www.livescience.com/43956-walking-10000-steps-healthy.html

Building and toning muscles

Walking builds and tones a surprising variety of muscles. Ankles, calves, quads, hamstrings, hips, gluts, abs and arms all get a workout when you walk.[3]

Preventing diabetes

A recent study done in Great Britain found that those who have a history of diabetes in their family saw an improved sensitivity to insulin when they added brisk walking into their routine.[4] Insulin resistance is associated with type II diabetes and heart disease. And a Harvard Nurses' Health Study found that walking for just 30 minutes a day cuts a woman's risk of type II diabetes by 30%.[5]

Stopping the meds

Using the data provided by the National Walkers' Health Study of over 32,000 women as well as 8000 men, researchers found that those who took longer walks each week were able to reduce the amount of diabetic, blood pressure and cholesterol medication they needed to manage their symptoms. The distance that they walked did not seem as important as how long they walked.[6]

Relieving pain

People who suffer from the chronic pain and fatigue of fibromyalgia reported marked relief after just a couple of weeks of moderate walking, according to a 2007 study.[7] It can also relieve lower back pain by loosening tight muscles, improving circulation,

---

[3] http://health.howstuffworks.com/wellness/diet-fitness/information/walking-to-lose-weight4.htm

[4] http://www.rodalenews.com/benefits-walking

[5] http://www.prevention.com/fitness/fitness-tips/healthiest-walking-workout-diabetics

[6] http://www.ncbi.nlm.nih.gov/pmc/articles/PMC3640497/

[7] http://www.webmd.com/fibromyalgia/features/exercise-can-ease-fibromyalgia-pain

and strengthening surrounding muscles, according to Dr. Grant Cooper, MD.[8]

Reducing your risk of a stroke

The stronger your heart is, the less likely you are to have a stroke. A study done at the University of South Carolina showed that walking briskly for only 30 minutes for five days a week lowers the risk of stroke by 40%.[9]

Boosting the immune system

Walk and stay well! According to Linda J. Vorvick, MD, walking boosts the immune system by cleaning out the lungs so you don't get sick, increasing the white blood cells which detect infection, and raising body temperature which kills bacteria.[10]

Reducing stress

Taking a nice walk, even for just 30 minutes is enough to reduce a lot of the stress that you are going through during the day. An Australian study found that walking after intense stress significantly reduced cortisol levels and improved the subjects' moods.[11] Incidentally, lots of experts, including Jillian Michaels, believe that high cortisol levels prevent the body from losing weight.[12] On those days when nothing is going right, and you are about to go crazy, taking a little walk around the block can be just reset button you need.

---

[8] http://www.spine-health.com/video/video-why-exercise-important-lower-back-pain

[9] http://www.rodalenews.com/benefits-walking

[10] http://www.nlm.nih.gov/medlineplus/ency/article/007165.htm

[11] http://www.sciencedirect.com/science/article/pii/002239999290072A

[12] http://www.jillianmichaels.com/fit/lose-weight/belly-fat-and-cortisol-connection

Preventing dementia

A 13 year study following healthy older adults (the mean age at the beginning of the study was 78) found that those who walked from 6 to 9 miles a week were half as likely to suffer from the cognitive impairment that leads to dementia.[13] Just doing some simple walking, it does not even need to be fast, can help to keep your brain alert.

Preventing osteoporosis

Walking is a weight-bearing activity that is good for strengthening the bones. Just a simple walk each day is going to strengthen the bones and make them stronger and denser. It can also help you to avoid joint conditions like arthritis.[14]

Promoting creative thinking

"I would walk along the quais [sic] when I had finished work or when I was trying to think something out. It was easier to think if I was walking and doing something or seeing people doing something that they understood." So said Ernest Hemingway, in A Moveable Feast.

Many distinguished writers, Thoreau, Frost and Austen to name three more, were vocal about their passion for walking. Several prominent CEOs, Steve Jobs, and Mark Zuckerberg to name two, held walking meetings with their staff to stir up the mental juices. A recent Stanford study reported that there is a biological connection between walking and creative ideas. Researchers found that creative thinking (but not analytical thinking) exploded by an average of 60% when the thinker moved about.[15]

---

[13] http://www.neurology.org/content/early/2010/10/13/WNL.0b013e3181f88359.abstract?maxtoshow=&hits=10&RESULTFORMAT=&fulltext=Erickson&searchid=1&FIRSTINDEX=0&sortspec=date&resourcetype=HWCIT

[14] http://www.webmd.com/osteoporosis/features/exercise-for-osteoporosis

[15] http://news.stanford.edu/news/2014/april/walking-vs-sitting-042414.html

Losing Weight

And then there is the really big argument, the number one reason that "10,000 Steps" has become the new fitness buzzword. Weight loss.

Walking is an aerobic activity that promotes weight loss. Maximum results are achieved by walking briskly for at least 30 minutes, but you can still get some benefits from a slower walk if that is all you are able to do.

Depending on the amount of weight that you carry and how fast you are going, you can burn quite a few calories just by walking. A nice brisk walk a few times a week and you will have the moderate exercise that is recommended by the CDC. According to Courtenay Schurman, the author of *The Outdoor Athlete*, you should start out slow if you are not currently active and build up to something that is more vigorous.[16] Some walkers will choose a distance, and others will choose to walk for a certain amount of time. It is best if you are able to combine the two of these and also keep on a heart rate monitor so you can figure out how hard you are working and if you need to put in more effort.

The important thing that you will need to watch is the intensity of the exercise you are doing. While some health conditions can be assisted with a light walk around the block, if you want to lose weight, it is important that you get a fast or brisk walk in your day to burn the calories and fat for weight loss. Each person will be able to handle a different intensity, so pay attention to your heart rate. Keep the rate somewhere near 70 percent of the maximum heart rate. For those who do not have a heart rate monitor, staying in the range of "moderate" to "high" intensity using the "talk test" lets you know you are walking fast enough to burn off those pounds. Here is how to gauge the intensity results of the talk

---

[16] http://www.webmd.com/fitness-exercise/guide/walking-for-exercise

test according to Kate Crosby, co-founder of Walk with Attitude & Pedometers Australia:[17]

Mild-you can chat away without any change in your breathing

Light-talking takes a bit of an effort, but it is still comfortable

Moderate-after every few words you need to take a breath

High-you cannot hold a conversation

Uncomfortable-gasping for breath (note: this is bad, take a break)

Being consistent and walking for at least 30 to 45 minutes at a moderate to high intensity is key to losing weight. But don't lose heart if you are not there on day one. Work into it, and keep it fun.

Lowering Blood Pressure

For those suffering from high blood pressure, it is critical that you are able to find effective ways to lower that number to improve the health of your heart. Lowering your blood pressure is not always as easy as you would think and sometimes even after exercise, eating right, reducing sodium, and taking medications the number is still going to be higher than you would like. Walking may be the solution that you have been looking for.

A study that was in the *Journal of Epidemiology and Community Health* looked at whether walking could lower blood pressure, and if so, how much was required for results. In this 12 week study of sedentary government workers, one-third of the participants were asked to walk briskly for 30 minutes five days a

---

17 http://www.walkingwithattitude.com/blog/how-to-use-the-talk-test-to-measure-your-walking-intensity/

week. A second group were asked to do the same thing, but only for three days a week. The final third were instructed to not change their lifestyles at all. All of the participants wore pedometers. At the beginning and end of the study, researchers recorded the waist size, hip measurement, overall fitness, weight, blood cholesterol, and blood pressure of the participants.

The results showed that the blood pressure dropped, as well as the waist and hip sizes, in the two groups who walked. This is good news when it comes to lowering your blood pressure because a few points can make a huge difference. This small decrease is enough to help reduce the risk of developing heart disease. This study also shows that any amount of exercise can be beneficial as the three-day walkers had almost the same benefits as the five-day walkers. And the walking doesn't even need to happen all at once. Three ten minute walks are effective. Not surprisingly, the control group did not see any changes at all.[18]

Better Mood

Feeling depressed, stressed out, or just down in the dumps? Everyone has those days, some more than others, and it can be difficult to get out of the slump. But studies have shown that getting up and moving is the perfect thing to do in order to improve your mood.

A study done at the University of Texas looked at those with serious depressive disorders to see which was more effective in helping their condition; either walking for 30 minutes on the treadmill or resting quietly on their own. At the end of the study, both of the groups reported better moods, but those who did the walking on the treadmill tended to feel more positive as well as having more energy.[19]

---

[18] http://www.webmd.com/hypertension-high-blood-pressure/news/20070815/a-little-walking-cuts-blood-pressure

[19] http://walking.about.com/od/mindandspirit/a/mood122005.htm

Even if you are not dealing with depression, you can take a walk in order to improve your mood. It is easy to do and as long as the walk is brisk and gets your heart rate up, it is possible to get the mood-boosting benefits.

These are just a few of the benefits that you can get from adding in 10,000 steps to your day. Even if you are not able to get up to this number each day, work toward it and you will find that the extra work is helping your heart.

So how can you tell what your current activity level is, and measure any improvements? The next chapter walks through different methods and gadgets for tracking your steps.

Chapter 2: Counting Your Steps

> "Phileas Fogg, having shut the door of his house at half-past eleven, and having put his right foot before his left five hundred and seventy-five times, and his left foot before his right five hundred and seventy-six times, reached the Reform Club"-Jules Verne, Around the World In 80 Days

Unless counting every step you take is one of the ways you keep those head screws tightened down (and we all do something), you are going to want a more sophisticated way to track your progress. Some people do this by setting a number of dedicated minutes for walking each day, or heading down a trail that is a known number of miles. The disadvantage of these solutions is that you don't get credit for waking into the kitchen for those eight daily glasses of water. And if you don't track those steps, you won't go out of your way to increase them, thereby missing out on scores of chances each day to burn extra calories and build muscle. Just by consciously tracking your steps, the process becomes a self-fulfilling path to success.

There are three main categories of devices that serve a pedometer function. Some are straight forward, some come with more bells and whistles than a fire department. They come in three basic categories: basic pedometers, health gadgets, and apps. Here is a look at how they can help you reach your goals.

Using a Pedometer

The pedometer is the most basic of the tools that you can use to make your new goal of 10,000 steps, but it is very effective and for many people it is all that they need to get motivated. Basic pedometers start a just a few dollars (though you can spend a few hundred or even a few thousand if you wish) and clip on to your shoe or belt. They have in a built-in accelerometer that is sensitive to the side-to-side motion you make when you walk, so don't put it in your pocket or purse. Some only track your steps, but some convert that distance into miles and calories too. Read the instructions (or just randomly push lots of buttons) to set it up and input whatever might be required for the internal calculations, like your weight or your stride length.

Using a step-counter or a pedometer is easy, and it can even be fun to keep track of all the activity that you are getting in. You will be able to add up each of the steps that are taken as long as you put it on right away in the morning. You can count all of the steps, your workouts, and all of the movement you are doing in order to get a good count by the end of the day.

You can also use the pedometer as a way to motivate yourself to get up and walk around some more. We all get lazy and feel like we have done enough. You can check the pedometer and see if you really did all of the work that you thought or if there are still more steps you need to get in order to reach your goal. This is a great motivator and will make sure you are up and moving as much as you need to be healthy.[20]

If your pedometer doesn't keep a daily log, it is a good idea to keep one by hand, or spreadsheet, or by plugging it into your computer if that is an option. It is hard to really appreciate your progress over time without the data, and also hard to know when it is time to start stretching your goals. It is also easier for you to distinguish patterns, like consistently falling short of your goal or surpassing it on particular days of the week. When you have the numbers, you can analyze them and interpret them, and understand your own needs a little better.

---

[20] http://www.webmd.com/fitness-exercise/using-a-pedometer-or-step-counter

Of course, you can always invest in a fancy gadget that will do a lot of the analysis for you, and a whole lot more.

Gadgets for Tracking Fitness

Pedometers are not the only way to monitor your steps throughout the day. There are some really cool products that you can check out. These devices are meant to not only motivate you, but to give you as much data as possible, and to help you set goals. Please note that I am not endorsing any of these products, nor have I actually used any of them. I am providing this list because I was curious as to what out there, and this is what I found. This is not a complete list of the products available either. I'd love to hear reader opinions. Also, note that all of these gadgets integrate with a variety of popular apps.

FitBit

The Fitbit Flex is most popular workout wristband in the marketplace at the time of this writing. It fits like a watch, comes in 10 different colors, tracks steps, distance, calories, and active minutes. It also tracks how long and well you sleep, and will wake you up with a vibration alarm. It has a display on the gadget, and also synchs up with your smartphone or computer so you can see your progress on the app of your choice. Their own app lets you also track calories consumed. FitBit has other products as well, from pedometers to gadgets that record your heart rate too.[21]

Nike+ Fuelbands

Nike has several different wristband products that are designed to monitor whole body movement, along with steps. They track your progress with Nike's own metric system, NikeFuel, instead of with calories burned. Points are awarded independent of weight or sex and are displayed with colored LED lights. The Fuelband has a feature called "Win the hour" which is awarded

---

[21] http://www.fitbit.com

when the wearer is up and moving for at least five minutes that hour, a concept that has been expounded quite a bit recently for heart health. As of this printing, and to the best of my possibly flawed knowledge, the Nike+ Move app only works on iOS, but the device works with other apps too.[22]

BodyMedia FIT

BodyMedia (recently acquired by Jawbone) makes bands that are worn on the upper arm (instead of the wrist). They track activity and sleep, and their app lets you log the food you consume so you can tell if your calorie input or output is greater. The app is supposed to be one of the best, but it isn't free; it is sold by monthly subscription. BodyMedia's claim to fame is that they measure calories burnt more accurately than other devices because they sense sweat and body temperature as well as movement.[23] The reviews I have read of the product seem to feel that this advantage is significant.

Jawbone Up

Jawbone, which now owns BodyMedia has its own line of fitness trackers called Up. Without having ever tried it myself or spoken to anyone who has worn one, the UP3 looks like one of the least expensive models that also monitors heart rate, and they claim to do it more accurately. Jawbone also has the Move, which is one of the few trackers under $50. All of the Up trackers are designed to look more like jewelry than gadgets and do not have readouts on the trackers themselves. The Up app lets you input food consumed, but the bands work with many of the leading fitness tracker apps as well.

---

[22] http://www.nike.com/us/en_us/c/nikeplus-fuel

[23] http://www.bodymedia.com/

Microsoft Band

Microsoft came late to the party, but the device they released in late 2014 seems to have taken the best of the other devices and integrated everything. Step counter, GPS, heart rate monitor, sleep monitor, coffee maker...well, maybe not that last part. The bracelet has a very Microsoft looking interface that provides all kinds of data. Works with the Microsoft Health app, and lots of others too.

Garmin Vivo

I have a soft spot in my heart for Garmin. Years ago I bought one of their armbands with a GPS tracker for running, and I was really happy with the device. The thing I loved most was that it gave me a virtual running partner that I raced against. The device would update me with how many feet in front or behind me my partner was (he ran at a steady pace), and it motivated me to push myself. That said, when I look at the Garmin products versus the competition, I notice two things. The first is that the VivoFit 2 and the VivoSmart are the least expensive models which include a heart rate monitor that I have seen, by quite a margin. The second is that they are my least favorite esthetically of the group. They appear to do everything, though, count steps, calories, monitor sleep and tell you when to get up and move.

Striiv

This brand is not as well-known, but it has a loyal following. Their products are colorful and inexpensive. The functions seem to be on the more basic side, but they might offer a good entry point. I don't see that any of their product offer heart monitoring. Like all the other brands, Striiv has its own app, or you can use with your favorite.[24]

[24] http://www.striiv.com/

Withings

Withings has several products with unique features. The Activite Pop looks like a waterproof watch, but it tracks distance, calories, swimming and sleep, and you don't have to charge it (the website says the battery lasts about 8 months). The Activite is a sleeker dress watch version. The Pulse O2 is a band that does require charging and measures all the usual things including your blood oxygen level. The drawback is that the heart rate monitor is not continuous. You have to stop and use it to take your pulse if you want a reading.

Smartphone

You might find that your smartphone already has all the functionality you need. Many smartphones can track steps, and some even can measure your heart rate, (though not as conveniently as a band). Combine that with the power of the leading fitness apps, and it is likely you already have what you need to keep track of your steps, monitor weight loss and set goals. The drawback is that since you are not always wearing it, you might not receive full credit for all your effort.

A thing to keep in mind is that all of these options come with one inherent flaw: they are not especially accurate. Assume an error margin of 10% whenever you are tracking your steps. Your gadget might register moving your arm as a step, or it might not count a few if your movements are too subtle.

In the end, it comes down to features and price. Decide how much you are willing to spend. Then decide which features are the most important to you. Do you want GPS so you can find your way home when taking new trails? To you want a heartrate monitor? Do you want to keep track of your sleep? Then read lots of product reviews (I use Amazon because they always have the volume) before making your decision. Sometimes a reviewer will bring up a point like, "sunscreen eats through the plastic" that might not be a deal breaker for you once you know about it, but it is something you need to know.

Once you find your gadget, you need to download the right app.

Walking Apps

You could track all your mileage in a good old-fashioned notebook, or on a spreadsheet. Those both work just fine. But there are a lot of fancier, and dare I say it, more fun, ways to keep track of your steps.

The first place to start is with the app that comes with your fitness band, if you have one, or with your smartphone. The reasons? You know they are compatible, and they won't have pop-up ads. Check it out, see how you like it. Is it easy to use, or too complicated? Does it show you what you want to know, or everything but? Do you have to manually start the app, or is it recording all the time? If you get a good fit straight out of the box, great! You are good to go. But if not, or maybe even in addition to it, you may want to look at what else is on the market.

If you open up the app store on your device, you will find thousands of fitness apps. Which ones do you look at? Some are great for CrossFit or weight training work outs. There are apps for just abs and just squats. Some track many different types of activity. Some incorporate diet as well. And some apps are made for walking. If you want an app to help keep track of your walks, check out some of these.

Charity Miles - Free

Charity Miles is a way to raise money for a charity of your choice (from a pretty robust list). When you are heading out for a bike ride, run, or walk, you activate this free app, select your charity, and start earning 0.10 a mile for biking, and 0.25 for each mile on foot. There is an additional $1.00 incentive for sharing a picture. You only need to walk 1/10 of a mile for the event to count. The app strongly encourages you to share your good work on social media, but for all who like to keep yourselves to yourselves, it is not strictly required. It works in conjunction with other apps and devices, so you can still count Charity Miles toward your daily goal.

Map My Walk – Free or Paid

Map My walk uses GPS tracking to record your walks, which is great for people like me who get lost somewhat regularly. It measures calories burned based on not just distance, but also elevation and pace. It tracks miles or kilometers instead of steps. It integrates with many of the most popular devices and phones, and also with other apps that are tracking steps. It even tells you when to buy new shoes.

Instant Heart Rate - Free

Instant Heart Rate uses the camera on your phone to measure your heart rate.

Pedometer - Free

A basic Pedometer app for smartphones that users seem to feel works reliably.

Runtastic – Free or Paid

Runtastic has similar features to Map My Walk. It measures distance in miles or kilometers, calculates calories based on distance, pace, and elevations, and uses a GPS to show you where you are and where you have been. It has a voice coach to encourage you and lets your friends cheer you on. It integrates with several music apps.

My Fitness Pal – Free

A really good app for logging food. Their website http://www.myfitnesspal.com/apps has links to various fitness apps and activity trackers, so it is a good place to do some exploring.

New apps are created every day. Old apps are updated all the time. Keep exploring and trying different ones until you find something that you really like.

Apps aren't just useful for tracking your walks; they can also provide great entertainment while you are out getting your exercise. Chapter four discusses ways to make walking more entertaining. But first, the next section covers ways to integrate more steps into your routine every day.

Chapter 3: Incorporating More Steps into Your Day

> "Everywhere is walking distance if you have the time"
> Stephen Wright

When you first get started, you may be discouraged by the number of steps you currently take every day. Most people walk 5000 or less. This does not mean that adding more steps into your life is going to be difficult. It will, however, need to be a consistent, gradual effort. You will need a plan, persistence, and some creativity in order to do it.

Before you start, wear the pedometer or gadget around for a few days. Do not do anything extra, just stick with the normal routine that you are already used to. Keep this up for a week and track the numbers that you have. This is your starting point and can give you a good idea of if you are close to your goal or if you still have quite a ways to go. You can also decide if you want to go for the full 10,000 steps or if you want to start slowly building up to that over time.

Now that you have a good idea of where you are starting, it is time to start incorporating more steps into your day. Here are ways to get more steps into the day without having to try too hard:

Wear comfortable shoes

You don't need to wear sneakers to the office, but investing in a good pair of shoes that are kind to your feet can make all the difference in walking more. If my feet hurt, not only do I not walk extra, I roll around in my office chair and try to avoid walking at all. I also keep a pair of sneakers in the car for running errands and walking when the chance presents itself.

Pace yourself

Instead of sitting or standing still, pace a bit. This can work no matter where you are at and provides you with lots of small workouts. I pace while talking on the phone, watching television, and while waiting for appointments, just walking back and forth to increase my steps. As a bonus, I always get right in to see the dentist.

Take the stairs

You don't have to take all the stairs at once. Start with one flight, and catch the elevator on the second floor. Take the stairs down, if your knees and joints give you permission. Going down might be less work, but it comes with its own kind of trouble, so go slow. You can take the stairs instead of the escalator too, or walk up the moving stairs instead of riding them.

Park further away

Parking in the back of the lot has lots of advantages. I increase my steps. Twice. I am less likely to get a door ding or have a shopping cart bump into my 2002 Subaru. I can find my car more easily. I am less likely to have an irritating driver wait for me to unload my groceries and drive away so they can take my spot. (Drivers that never read the articles which say that people take longer to move when you are waiting for them). And when I walk my cart back to the store instead of the cart return, I double my parking lot steps.

Do an extra lap at the store

After parking further away at the store, sometimes I do a victory lap around the store perimeter before I check out. Sometimes I see items I forgot to put on my list.

Stroll while your wait

My kids are on a swim team which practices at the local college. Unfortunately, they are too young to drive, so my wife and I switch off playing chauffeur. While they are doing their laps, I stroll around the campus listening to a book. I stop and get a coffee. I make it back in time to see their progress and chat with other parents.

Sometimes, when I'm early to appointments, I walk around the block instead of reading a magazine in the waiting room.

Walk to work

I walk to and from work every single day. Given that I work from home, the seven-second commute doesn't really rack up many steps. But, if you are lucky enough to live within a mile or two from work, you can get your 10,000 steps in and de-stress. If you take public transportation, consider getting on or off a stop early, and walking an extra few blocks. Little workouts add up.

Go out to lunch

The healthiest and most budget friendly option is usually to bring lunch from home. If you do (and well done you!), instead of eating at your desk, find a place where you can eat out of doors when the weather is nice. Soak up the vitamin D. Take a walk around the block when you are done. When the weather is bad, eat in a break room and walk the stairs. You get a break and some steps at the same time. If you don't bring your lunch, switch it up and walk to get lunch instead of ordering in. A clear and fresh head most likely means you'll be more productive when you return. You can also leave the office for a coffee break and walk around the block. If you want to score brownie points, offer to go get your boss an Americano.

Move throughout the day

In another lifetime, I used to work in sales. There was a guy in my office, who every hour, on the hour, got up from his desk and walked out the door. Fifteen minutes later he walked back in. For the first week on the job, I assumed he was a smoker. I resented the fact that his filthy disgusting habit (I had quit the year before) allowed him to work 25% less than everyone else. And one day I cleverly found out by making self-righteous comments to the receptionist that 1. He was out walking, and 2. His sales figures were among the highest in the office. By clearing his head every hour, he was able to focus more productively the rest of the time.

Not everyone has a boss who will let them skip out for a quarter of the day every day though the world might be a healthier place if they did. Research shows that sitting for prolonged periods can restrict your blood flow, which contributes to heart disease. You can avoid or even reverse this damage by frequently moving throughout the day.[25] So be creative if you must. Set the alarm on your fitness band, or better yet, drink lots of water. If you can use a restroom on another floor, you take more steps. Instead of calling or emailing colleagues, walk over to their desk. You save the time that comes with the back and forth and waiting involved in written communication, and you get the added benefit of watching them rush to close that Candy Crush window.

Go to the park

Parks are great for kids and dogs, but they are adult approved as well. If do have a child or a canine who you can take with you, so much the better! I know parents who use the playground as a gym, getting upper body workouts on the monkey bars and doing box jumps on the benches. I am less ambitious. But I get steps in while my kids ride their bikes on the way there and back, and I walk the path or track while they shove each other off of the swings.

---

[25] http://www.washingtonpost.com/news/to-your-health/wp/2014/09/08/take-a-seat-you-may-be-able-to-reverse-the-damage-to-your-health/

Take a turn after dinner

Especially during the spring and summer when it stays lighter longer, taking a stroll after dinner is a great way to digest your food, and maybe even connect with your family if you can drag them along. You can go around the block once, or several miles as you like, and you won't be tempted by the cookie jar if it isn't in front of you. One word of caution, dusk and dawn are the perfect times to be consumed wholly by mosquitos during certain times of the year. Wear long sleeves and trousers if you live in a mosquito-y area.

Walk and Watch (Television)

A friend of mine believes that if all televisions were powered via treadmill, we wouldn't have a weight problem in this country. I'm envisioning all the hospital (and perhaps vet) visits that would result from people with "great ideas". Regardless, there's no denying that it is tempting to end the night by watching your favorite television show or three and doing nothing else. The day at work can get to you, and you might want just to unwind and relax. But just staring at the television at night is bad for your health; first, if you sit around after a hearty dinner, those calories aren't getting used, and second, there are pizza commercials. To make this experience more health friendly, turn it into a workout. Each time a commercial comes on, get up and pace. Even better, see if you can jog in place for the few minutes to get the heart pumping, or do squats, or sit-ups. It is only a few minutes here and there, but for an hour program you can end up with over 20 minutes of workout that you would not have had otherwise. If you are streaming shows sans commercials, pause the show between scenes every once in a while, or when someone watching the show with you starts to talk. Ahem. Or watch it part of it on a treadmill.

Tramp to your errands

I'm fortunate enough that I live in a town that is so small; I can walk to the market, the library, and the post office in under 20 minutes. I'll admit that sometimes I don't, because I'm feeling lazy or rushed, or it is snowing or I'll have my hands full. But when I make myself walk those errands, I'm always glad I did, and I'm more likely to walk them the next time.

March your kids to school

If you live close enough to walk the kids to school, they learn the route and get a better understanding of the neighborhood, and you get to smirk at all the moms and dads waiting in the kiss-and-go drop off line. It feels even better when you have the dog and a mug of coffee.

Switch out happy hour for a hike

Instead of meeting friends after work for a cocktail, take a walk with them instead. You save twice; the calories and the cash. You can substitute a saunter for a lavish lunch as well.

Mosey the mall

There are lots of reasons people prefer to do their walking indoors instead of outside. Weather, safety concerns, car exhaust, and uneven terrain can make walking outside a non-starter. Fortunately, many malls have indoor walking programs, where they open the doors early so people can get their exercise for the day.[26] Malls are great for walking. You can do one lap or twenty. You can find a friend to talk to, or silently race "that one guy". You can window shop. If your local mall doesn't have a formal program, you can walk there during business hours.

Geocache

There are millions of geocaches hidden around the world. All you need is an app to look for them. Geocaching is treasure hunting for small treasures that other people have hidden. You find them purely for bragging rights. It is fun, frustrating, rewarding, and highly addictive. Chances are, there are several geocaches within walking distance of your house. It is a great activity to do by

---

[26] http://www.prevention.com/fitness/fitness-tips/mall-walking-tips

yourself, or with the whole family (but watch out for muggles!) To learn more, check out https://www.geocaching.com/play.

Tour the town

Walking tours are guided, or self-guided, walks through an area, usually designed to highlight the history of the place. They can be a great way to get to see a new city, or even to get reacquainted with your hometown. They can be led by a formal guide, or you can purchase or download instructions to follow yourself.

The first walking tour I remember taking was part of a package my wife and I bought for our first anniversary. We went to San Francisco at the last minute and wanted to see Alcatraz, but didn't book it in advance and the whole weekend was sold out. We had to buy tickets through a "broker" (AKA guy on the street) who justified his mark-up by bundling them with a historic tour of San Francisco a pied. He walked like a bullet train, and I'm pretty sure that he made up quite a bit of his "history", but it didn't matter. We were hooked.

Since then, we have taken walking tours all over, alone and with the kids. Underground Seattle (the guides are hilarious!), Jane Austen's Bath, and an architecture tour of Chicago are the ones that stand out in my memory. Most cities and even neighborhoods have some kind of a walking tour where you can get history and steps at the same time. Some places have apps you can download, or phone numbers posted throughout the town to call to hear history recordings.

Great places to find about walking tours are guidebooks, visitor centers, or my favorite way to find anything, googling it on the internet.

Hit a museum

Museums are fantastic places to walk because they have so much to look at while you are doing it. Art museums, history museums, science museums, all have something rewarding to offer. Visit each one in your town, and then become a member of your favorite. You get invited to new exhibits first, and many museums have reciprocal privileges with other museums when you travel.

Walk a trail

And last, but not least, is my very favorite; the traditional scenic walk. I live in an area where there are lots of beautiful trails, but I especially appreciate scenic walks when I'm visiting somewhere new. I like walking through older or grander neighborhoods and checking out the houses. I like getting away from suburban traffic in an open space. I like checking out the shops and restaurants in urban areas. And, of course, there's the quintessential walk on the beach.

It isn't always easy to know where to walk when you are traveling. I was fortunate enough to visit Israel once. I stayed in a hotel and wanted to walk around after dinner, so I asked the (armed) guard at the door if the neighborhood was safe. He said it was, but then as I began walking down the street he called after me, "Unless you are unlucky." I didn't know what that meant, but I didn't test my luck very long.

I have had good luck in the US recently with a website called traillink.com. When you click on the state, it gives you a list of alphabetized trails, which isn't so helpful. If you click on the green "View results on Map" button at the top of the page, you can put in a city or zip code, and see the trails in a more meaningful way. Then you can click on the trail for more information, like distance, the type of terrain, difficulty, etc. It is good for bike trails too.

There is a similar map for national trails in the UK though I've never used it personally, at http://www.gps-routes.co.uk/routes/home.nsf/walking-routes-on-national-trails and one for Australia at http://www.australia.com/en/itineraries/walking-australia.html.

Chapter 4: Making it Fun

> "I breathe, I walk, I listen, I love. But not in that order, because right now I'm sitting down, testing my lung's storage capacity, and ignoring you."
> — Jarod Kintz, Love quotes for the ages. And the ageless sages.

Habit can be comforting, but walking the same route day after day to the last syllable of recorded time gets tedious. If you are anything like me, the more chore-like my routine becomes, the more inventive are my excuses not to do it. I need motivation.

Fortunately, there are lots of ways to spice up a walk. Each person will have different ideas of what will make the walk more fun, but once you discover what works for you, it can become positively addicting. Here are some of my favorites:

Listen to Something You Enjoy

Music, podcasts, audiobooks...listening while you walk can transport you, rejuvenate you, and turn your walk into your favorite time of the day.

The easiest way to take the sounds with you is on a smartphone, mp3 player, or some kind of small smart device. If you are in the minority of adults who don't have a smartphone yet, you can find an mp3 player to fit any budget if you shop around online.

Music

If you have uploaded your music collection already, you are good to go. Make an energetic playlist that is as broad as you can get it, and shuffle before you walk. Older music tape players, CD players, and radio headsets work fine too.

If you don't already have a digital musical library, there are several apps, both free and through a subscription that you can use to listen to the tunes you like. You create your own station built around a musical genre or artist, and it can be as mainstream or as specific as you like. Build a station around Beethoven's Ninth, 1960s crooners, Fleetwood Mac, modern alternative music, or Tuvan Throat Singing as you like. If a free app has a paid version, the difference is usually that the free version has commercials. Take a look at Pandora (my favorite), Spotify, IHeartRadio, Google Play, iTunes Radio and Xbox Music.

The upside to streaming music is the variety. The downside is that it can eat through your phone's streaming minutes if you don't have a Wi-Fi connection on your walk. You might also not have a signal everywhere you go. For those reasons, I usually limit streaming music to when I'm indoors with Wi-Fi.

Podcasts

Podcasts are like downloading episodes of radio programs. Some are slick and professional; some are so organic you can smell the patchouli oil through the headphones. You can find a podcast series on virtually anything from politics to comedy (those are different) to DIY.

I'm a big public radio fan, and I really like the podcasts NPR puts out. You can find a directory at http://www.npr.org/podcasts/organizations/1. Here is another list of fun podcasts: http://www.slate.com/articles/arts/ten_years_in_your_ears/2014/12/best_podcast_episodes_ever_the_25_best_from_serial_to_the_ricky_gervais.html.

If you have an account with iTunes, Xbox, or Google Play, they have directories of their podcasts. My favorite are the old time radio rebroadcasts, like *The Shadow* and *The Whistler*. There are even apps with old time radio content. Look around until you find something that grabs you.

Audio Books

Audio books aren't nearly as popular as eBooks, and I'm not sure why. They are a great way to enjoy a book while you are doing something else, like driving or cooking or walking. They are usually read by professional actors and are very entertaining. They are also easy to find and download. I find I listen to more books than I read these days because I rarely make time to sit still with a book. I can also listen to audio books together with my wife or kids, and we can share the experience.

You can get audio books by subscription, on sites like Audible.com and iTunes. The advantage to these site is that they have a dizzying number of titles, all the latest best-sellers, and the titles are always available. The disadvantage? I am frugal, and I like to find things for free. I download 99% of all my audiobooks from the library.

When libraries first started with audio book downloads, the process was significantly harder than it is now. If fact, it was such a pain, fraught with so many opportunities for mishap, that a lot of users decided it wasn't worth it. If you were one of those users, let me assure you, it is a different world out there now.

To download books from your library, you need a library card, and an app called Overdrive Media Console, which you download from your app store. Once you download the app, you select your library from a list, input your library card number, and voila, you can download audiobooks (and eBooks too!) for free. The disadvantage to this method is that your library might not have the title you want, or it might be checked out by someone else and you have to wait, because libraries only are allowed to lend a title to so many people at once. I counter this by getting library cards wherever I can, and so have access to the collections of several libraries.

Many libraries still offer books on CD that you can listen to on a portable player, and "playaways," little mp3 players with just one book. Those are extremely limited, though, and getting rarer by the second.

When I am in the middle of a good book, I'll keep walking or make excuses to do activity just to finish listening to it. I'll also ignore my family to the point where my wife had to establish rules about audiobook etiquette in our family. Sigh. First world problems indeed.

Walk with a friend or club

Another way to make your exercise entertaining is to walk and talk with someone you like. Finding a partner also keeps you accountable and you are more likely to go when someone is relying on you. You can walk with a spouse or partner and make it a time to connect. You can walk with someone at the office during lunch or after work. You can walk with a neighbor or friend. A dog makes a reliable walking partner because they are so darn *persistent*. Or, you can join a walking club.

Walking clubs are groups that, well, walk. When you join a walking club, you get to meet new people. Members encourage each other. And you are not dependent on one other person to keep you going because friends and spouses and neighbors can have other priorities. When you walk with a group you get exposed to new routes, you have safety in numbers, and you have the wisdom and experience of the collective.

To find a walking group in your area:

One place to look is on meetup.com. Meetup.com is a worldwide site for all types of groups, from writing groups to winetasting events to fitness clubs. Put in your area and what you are looking for, and you'll see information about the groups that are around and who to contact to join. This article at http://walking.about.com/od/walkingclubs/a/walkingclub.htm also lists other options about where to find a club.

In the UK, you can also check out http://www.ramblingclubs.com/rambling.php, http://www.ramblers.org.uk/, http://www.ldwa.org.uk/, and http://www.walkingclub.org.uk/.

In Australia, also look at http://www.walkingsa.org.au/walk/list-of-walking-clubs-south-australia/, http://www.bushwalkingnsw.org.au/clubs/,

Train for an event

If you are a goal-oriented person, training for a specific event might help you push yourself harder. Many of the events for runners have walking waves as well. Get friend to sign up too, and train together! You can find events that range in distance from just a few miles to marathons and longer.

For a list of events in your area, check out http://www.active.com/walking. They list events all over the world. You could also find an event in a place you've always wanted to go, and make it a destination.

In our family, we have certain events we do every year with friends, and even the kids are involved now. Some of the traditions have become fairly grand over the years, with friends flying in from around the country. Traditionally, we participate in races for St. Patty's Day, the Boulder Bolder over Memorial Day, the Susan G Komen Race for the Cure in October, and a Turkey Trot on Thanksgiving. The smack talk and banter starts months ahead of time. And we follow up the races with barbecues and parties.

Make it a Competition

If you are the competitive sort, start or join a competition. You can set it up with friends or at work or in a club.

Competitions can be organized around a number of goals. Steps walked, pounds lost, time logged, whatever. Competitions are more attractive when there is a prize at the end, be it bragging rights, or a pool of money.

If you work for a large organization, you can pitch the idea to HR as a way to reduce costs associated with health care and sick time. You might even be able to get them to sponsor a prize.

For competition to be effective, you want the largest number of participants. If you can talk someone with a big ego and a bigger mouth into joining (your boss?), they can take care of the recruitment for you. Research shows that whatever people actually admit to, peer pressure (or herd mentality) is still way more effective at motivating behavior than an appeal to a sense of higher purpose.

Do you have any other tips for staying committed while walking toward your weight loss goals? I'd love to hear about them. In addition to staying motivated when you are on the trail, you also need to stay safe. That is where the next chapter comes in.

Chapter 5: Playing it safe

> "No one saves us but ourselves. No one can and no one may. We ourselves must walk the path."
> — Gautama Buddha, *Sayings of Buddha*

Beginning a walking program has so many benefits, but it is important that you take the time to be safe and not cause any injuries or harm while you are at it. Walking is generally safe for most people, regardless of their activity and fitness levels, but you should check with your doctor first before you start a program. And once you begin, there are still a few things you can watch out for to make sure that you stay safe and get the best workout possible.

Wear Good Walking Shoes

Before you start walking a lot, it is a good idea to make sure that you invest in a good pair of walking shoes. These can help you to stand straight, have good form, and will prevent you from twisting your ankle or stepping wrong. Proper fit can also provide comfort so your feet will not hurt when you are done.

Wearing the right shoes while walking is a fundamental part of preventing injuries and maximizing benefit. Think of your shoes as a tool for walking; with the proper pair you will be able to do almost anything. Picking out the right shoes can take some time, but after you figure out what works the best for you, it can become much easier. Here are a few things that you should look for in a good pair of shoes according to livestrong.com[27]

Match the shoes with your body

High arches? Flat feet? Pronated stride? Your feet could be causing the rest of your body to overcompensate, and you could end up feeling pain in the other parts; lower back, hips, knees, ankles, and heels. [28]

When you are not comfortable during a walk, you will not be able to go as far, as fast, or endure as well. You will not be likely to continue on with walking if you are feeling miserable, and when you are in pain, you will cut the workout short. Finding a good shoe that fits your own foot and is able to change up the pressure that you are exerting on the body will promote a better walking workout without any injuries.

Have your stride analyzed by personnel at a quality running store, and they can outfit you with the right shoes to help. Another option is to visit an expert in sports medicine or a podiatrist; they will take the time to determine the needs of your foot and which shoe will help you. If all else fails, try on a few pairs of shoes and walk around the store to see which one provides the best comfort, fit, and support.

Cost

Be prepared to pay for quality. Good shoes will cost more, but these walking shoes will be worth it. The support that you get will be great and you will be able to walk faster and go for longer. Think of the price as an investment to help you improve your health, perform better, and prevent injuries.

---

[27] http://www.livestrong.com/article/76043-important-wear-good-walking-shoes/

[28] http://www.makingstridz.com/node/66

Replacing the shoes

But nothing gold can stay, Ponyboy. The American Academy of Physical Medicine and Rehabilitation recommends that you replace your shoes around each six months, or about every 400 miles depending on how heavy of a walker you are[29]. Over time, the shoe is going to wear down and not be as effective. Waiting too long might cause you pain and increase your chances of injury.

Drink plenty of water

While you are out walking, it is critical that you drink plenty of water. Don't wait until you are thirsty. Drink up before you leave and often along the way. Your body is working hard. If it is sunny and hot out, you are probably losing fluids even faster as your body sweats to cool you down. Failure to bring water might result in the body getting overheated and dehydrated; in extreme cases you may pass out or become really sick.

Before you start regularly walking , think about what kind of water container works best for you. To you want a metal reusable bottle that stays cold? Disposable bottles you can recycle when they are empty? A hydration system that fits on your back or waist and leaves your hands free? Carrying a bottle gets on my nerves, so I use a Camelbak system. There are bottles that clip to your arms and belt as well, to keep your hands free. Walk around a sporting goods store and see what your choices are and what feels right to you. And if your pooch will be your partner, spring for a collapsible bowl for her too.

---

[29] http://www.aapmr.org/Pages/default.aspx

And then there is too much water...

The downside to staying hydrated is you might need a pit spot or two along the way. It happens to everyone. I try to notice places I pass that would be useful in such an event. A gas station here, a park facility there. When nature calls, don't let it go to voicemail.

Enjoying and avoiding the sun

Walking is a great way to soak up some sunshine and vitamin D, but your skin might not be able to go for long without getting burned. Be especially careful in new environments. Even in the winter, the sun's reflections off of the snow can scorch your face in no time. The same goes for reflections off the water. And just because it doesn't feel warm doesn't mean you aren't getting zapped by UV rays. Remember the walking tour of San Francisco I mentioned a few chapters ago? Worse sunburn I've ever had happened that day, and I had sunscreen in my backpack the entire time. I just never put it on because it wasn't hot.

Make it a routine to put sunscreen on your face, sunglasses with UV protection on your eyes and hat on your head before you walk out the door.

The Skin Cancer Foundation recommends covering your arms and legs as well to protect against the sun[30], but when you are doing intense walking, it can sometimes get too hot. Use sunscreen on any areas that will be exposed for long. Sunscreen protects against sunburns, wrinkles, and skin cancer. Some sunblock basics:

1. Choose a sunscreen that is waterproof (so that the sweat does not wash it off) and that is at least SPF 15.

---

[30] http://www.skincancer.org/

2. Apply it about 30 minutes before you go on the walk. This allows the skin to absorb the sunscreen for best protection.
3. Put the lotion on thickly.
4. Do not forget the ears, bald spots, and your feet if you are wearing footwear which exposes some skin.
5. Use some lip balm that has an SPF in it as well in order to protect your kisser.
6. Throw it in your backpack if you will be out all day.
7. Choose sunblock with insect repellent if you are in a place with mosquitos.

Tips for walking in safety

Let's be careful out there. It's as true on your street as on Hill Street. Some things to keep in mind:

1. Always bring your ID. In an emergency, you will need it. You will also need it if you stop for a beer.
2. Have a few dollars or a credit card on you. You might need them to buy a sports drink at the gas station after you use their facilities, or to call a cab to bring you home.
3. Bring your house key too, in case your spouse runs to the store while you are gone and locks that door you specifically left open.
4. Dress for the weather. If it is cold or rainy, remember the mantra "cotton kills." Wear synthetics, and dress in layers that you can shed when the activity starts to warm you.
5. Wear bright clothing so others can see you and something reflective at night. Lots of sports attire has reflective material sewn into it.
6. Have a keychain size flashlight with you. Because when you need a flashlight, you really need a flashlight.

7. Stay on a path. When you stray, you can damage wildlife, or it can damage you.
8. Watch for crazy drivers talking on cell phones. Having the right of way is a small comfort when you are in traction.
9. Walk with a companion. You are less vulnerable, and there is someone to help you if you twist an ankle.
10. Pay attention to your surroundings. Notice other people and landmarks. Channel your inner Jason Bourne.
11. Watch for uneven or slippery terrain.
12. Bring your cellphone. It can track your steps, provide your entertainment, and show you a map if you get lost. Oh, and it is a phone.

Being properly prepared takes only a minute or two of planning, but can make all the difference. Keep a small backpack or hip bag that holds your walking gear and a water bottle, and you are ready to step out at any time.

Conclusion

> "Now shall I walk or shall I ride?
> 'Ride,' Pleasure said;
> 'Walk,' Joy replied."
> — W.H. Davies, The Best Friend

Walking is a wonderful way to lose weight and ward of a host of illnesses and diseases. It conditions both the body and the brain and can provide time throughout the day for you to relax and regroup.

Walking 10,000 steps each day burns a significant number of calories. Steps can be taken in lots of mini workouts instead of all at once. Those who are not prepared to walk 10,000 steps tomorrow can walk what they can, and build to their goal. There is a variety of gadgets and apps to help you keep track of the number of steps you take and to help set your goals.

Adding steps in unexpected places, and keeping your fitness routine interesting are the keys in making walking 10,000 steps a habit for the long-term. Listening to something interesting, walking with others, and blazing new trails are ways to transform your workout from a burden into the favorite part of your day.

Being prepared and safe while you are walking is critical. Keep a pack with your walking gear ready to go.

Make walking a part of your holidays and vacations. Make it a part of the time you spend with your friends and family. Make it a time to spend alone. Make walking a part of your identity, and your health and your spirit will reward you.

Message from the Author

One of the reasons that I love researching and writing in the information age is that it is easier than ever to connect with readers. Many of you generously let me know about new data and studies when they first come available and even share with me your own personal stories. If you have tips to share, or a story about your success while walking that you think would help others, let me know! Please keep your comments coming. You can connect with me by email at ryanjsmartin@gmail.com, via twitter at @ryanjsmartin, or on my Facebook page.

If you'd like to help other readers decide if this book is for them, I'd be grateful if you could take a moment and post a sentence or two as a review. Reader comments are the most powerful and unbiased way for others to determine which books should make the short list for their next read.

To your health,

Ryan

FREE DOWNLOAD

25 EASY HABITS

TO LIVE LONGER, HEALTHIER, AND HAPPIER

Bright Ideas Editoria

RYAN J. S. MARTIN

As a way of thanking you for purchasing this book, I am offering a special gift to my readers. This book is not available for purchase anywhere. You can only get it by clicking on the link below.

The power of habit is life altering. Smaller habits are easier to start and stop, and they can have measurable effects in the quality of a person's life. Smaller habits, once formed, grow into larger ones.

Habits can affect your body, your mind, and your spirit. They govern your interactions with friends and family. They control how you work and play. They form the basis for your success and failures.

Whether you have big changes you are ready to make in your life or just want to fine-tune small behaviors, this book can make a difference.

You can download the free book at https://editoria.leadpages.net/25habits/

Other Books by Ryan J. S. Martin

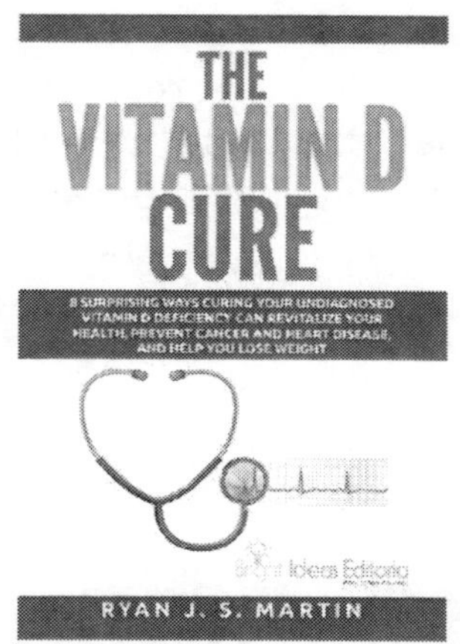

The Vitamin D Cure: 8 Surprising Ways Curing Your Undiagnosed Vitamin D Deficiency Can Revitalize Your Health, Prevent Cancer and Heart Disease, and Help You Lose Weight

Are you getting enough of the "miracle vitamin"? More than a billion people in the world today suffer from a moderate to severe Vitamin D deficiency – and they don't even know it! The Vitamin D Council in the US links Vitamin D deficiency to no fewer than 45 different diseases and conditions, from acne to tuberculosis. Can adding a Vitamin D supplement supercharge your immune system and improve the way you feel every day? Can eating a Paleo Diet make you more or less susceptible a range of diseases? Can spending a little time in the sun strengthen your bones, and help you to lose weight? Take control of your body and begin feeling great as you participate in The Vitamin D Cure!

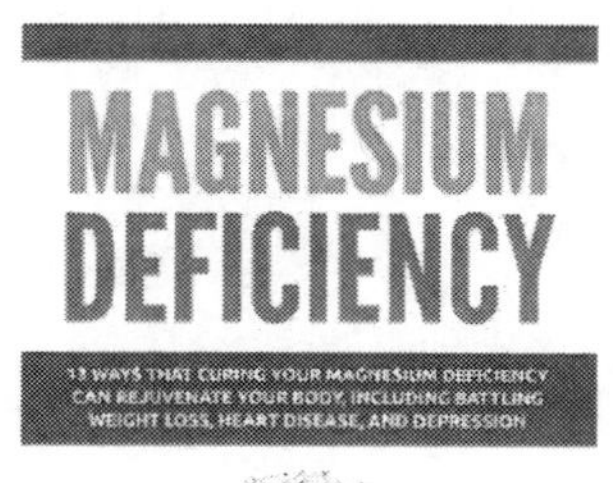

Magnesium Deficiency Magnesium Deficiency: Weight Loss, Heart Disease and Depression, 13 Ways that Curing Your Magnesium Deficiency Can Rejuvenate Your Body

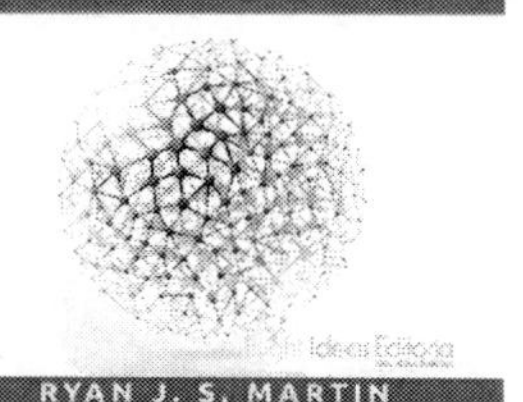

More than 300 processes in the body, including burning fat, converting sugar into energy, relaxing muscles, falling asleep, and just feeling happy, are all, in one way or another, regulated by magnesium. More than half of Americans and some estimates put this number at as high as 80%, don't get enough of this powerful mineral every day. This deficiency causes all sorts of problems with our muscles, bones, nerves, and brains. Doctors who have studied magnesium feel that we are just beginning to get an idea of what this mineral is responsible for, and how it can help treat and prevent disease. Get the facts, and learn what you need to know to prevent and treat a variety of health conditions with the "miracle mineral."

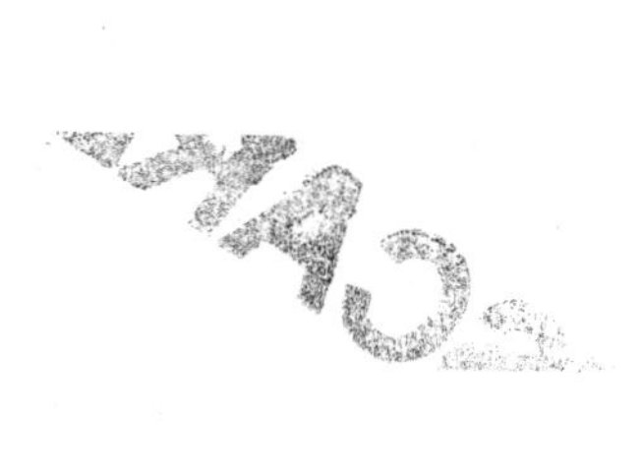

CPSIA information can be obtained at www.ICGtesting.com
Printed in the USA
LVOW10s1138080615

441602LV00002B/343/P